Squat Everyday for Kettlebell
8 Week Program
Bonus 6 Week Olympic Lifting Program

Designed and written by Douglas Seamans Jr

Owner and Head Instructor – PRIDE Conditioning

2015 AKA Nationals 1st Place & North American record Long Cycle - 85kg lifter – 28kg
2015 IUKL European Championships 1st place Long Cycle – 95kg lifter – 24kg
2015 IUKL World Championships 5th place - 95kg lifter – 24kg
2016 IUKL World Championships 3rd place - 95kg lifter – 24kg
2017 IUKL World Championships 2nd place - 95kg lifter – 24kg
2015 AKA Nationals 1st Place – 95kg lifters - 32kg

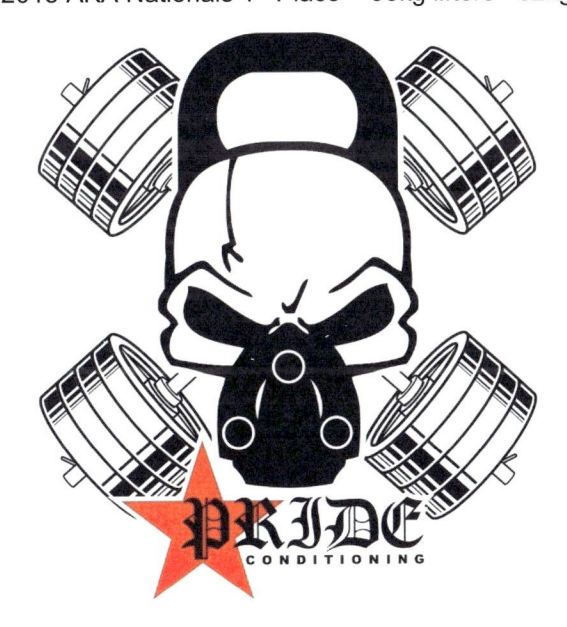

PRIDE Conditioning – 337 Dalton Ave, Charlotte, NC 28206

Please visit our website and blog for workouts, articles, training tips, motivation and recipes:
WWW.PRIDECONDITIONING.COM

Please visit our Youtube channel for videos on workouts and training tips:
http://www.youtube.com/user/PRIDECONDITIONING

This book is NOT for beginner lifters!

If you do not know how to use a kettlebell, how to squat, how to deadlift, how to do a clean and jerk on a barbell or with a kettlebell, and if you have never competed in a kettlebell lifting competition this book is NOT for you!

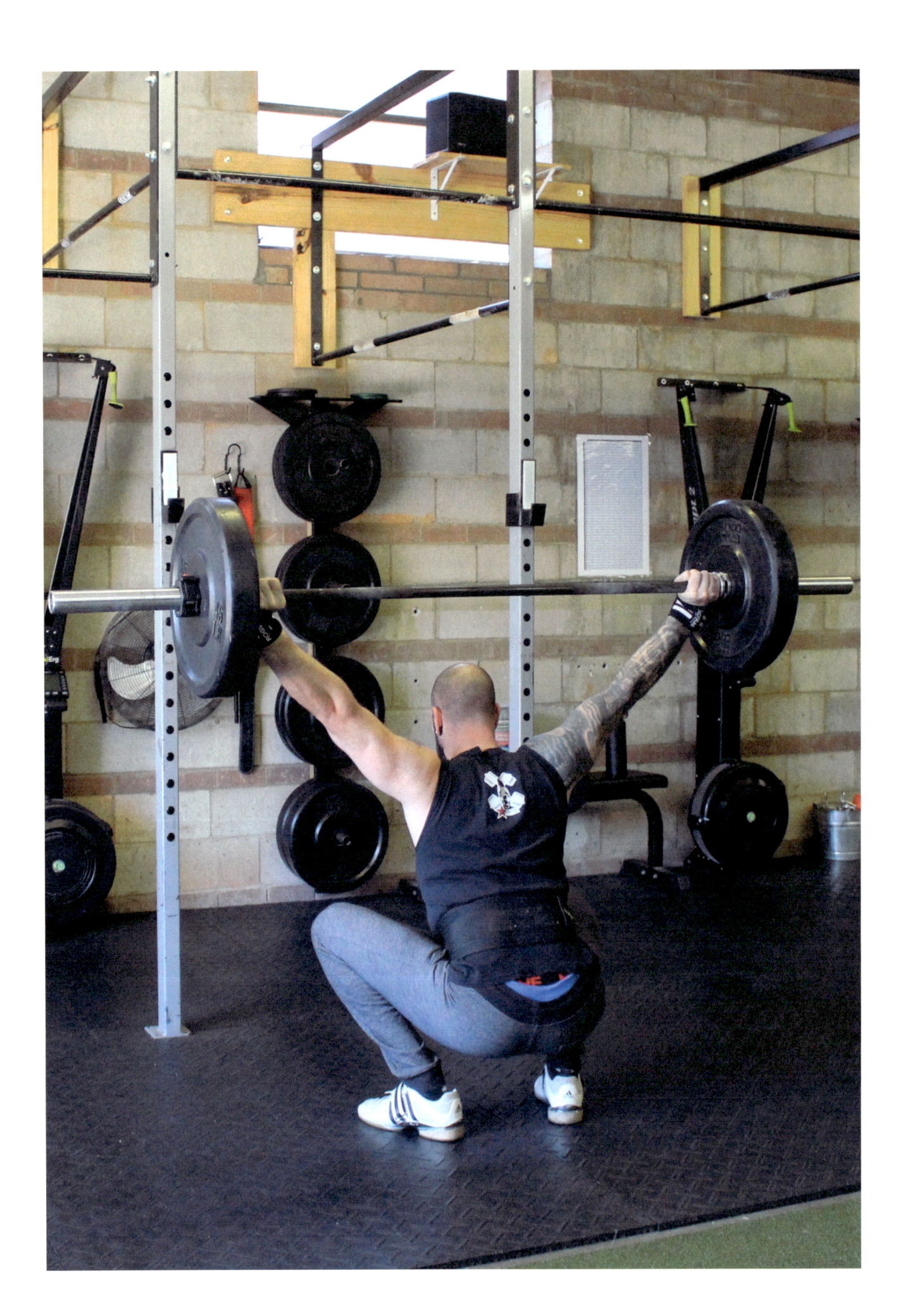

The information in this manual is copyrighted and is the sole legal property of PRIDE Conditioning and Douglas Seamans and is not to be shared or distributed without permission from the owner and publisher.

Dedication

This book is dedicated solely to my wife Lindsay. Lindsay and I have been through good and bad and all of our journeys and adventures and all the tough times and happy times have made us stronger. Lindsay has stood behind me and supported me through every endeavor, the gym, the apparel business, training to fight, training to compete in kettlebell, building hotrods, and all the traveling the world. I am thankful to have married someone I can truly call my best friend. Thank you for all your support and help wifeola, I could not have done any of this without you.

"Marriage is a never ending sleepover with your favorite weirdo!"

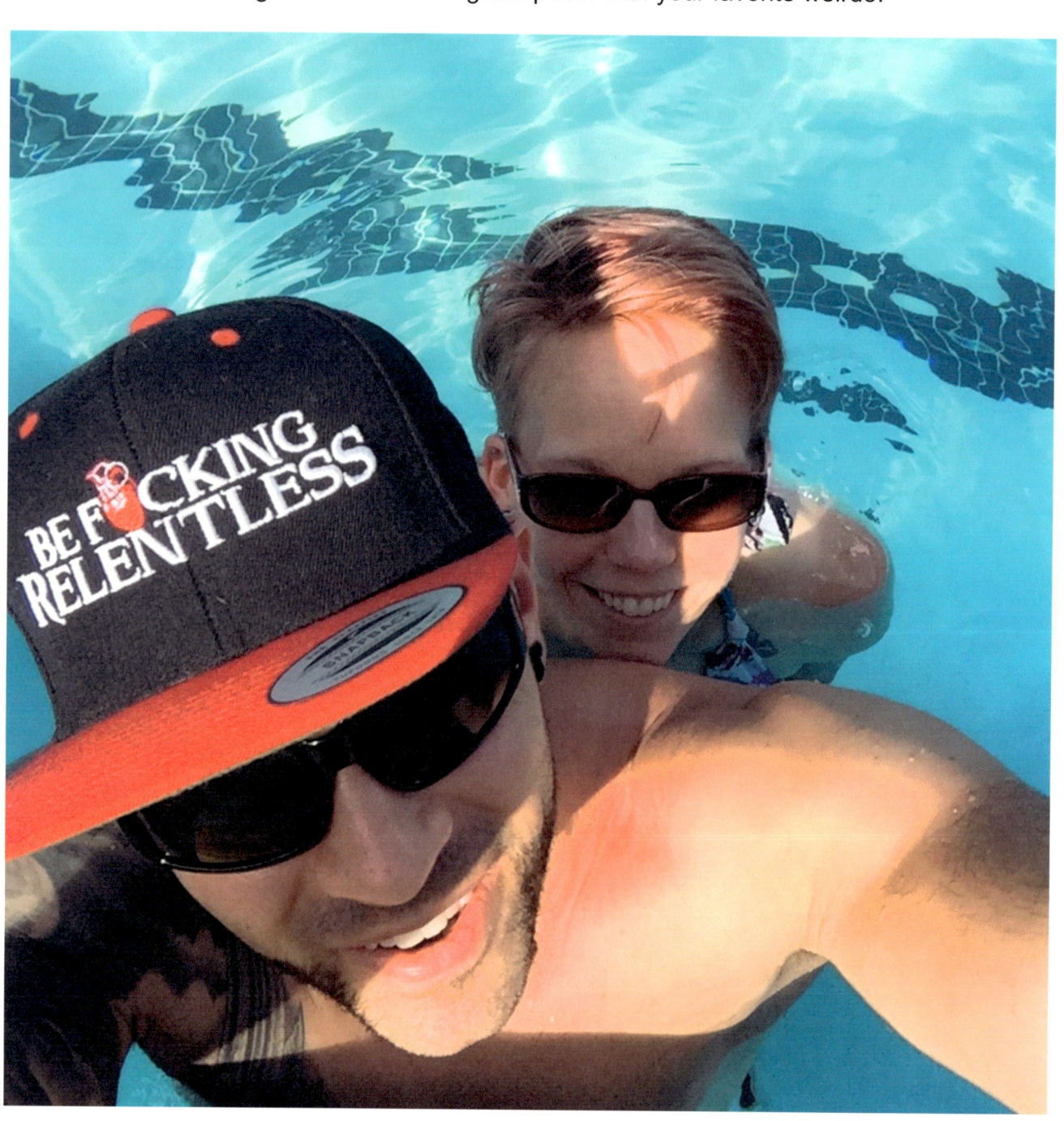

Introduction

This program can be done as a two a day routine, or the squats can be done as your warmup for your kettlebell sets (that is how I did it). If you choose to do a two a day program, squats in the morning and kettlebell or cardio in the evening you will be fine, the squats should only take you 30 minutes to complete. The type of squats chosen for this program are chosen specifically for kettlebell sport and all are chosen for specific reasons. We do front squats because it is more quad dominant and the weight is on the front of your body just like doing jerks, back squats and paused back squats for overall strength, box squats with chains for more explosive power, cleans to promote speed and power, and overhead squats to promote mobility and to strengthen the shoulders and upper back.

From novice to advanced, almost everyone can use this program! As long as you can squat and you have the mobility for overhead squats this program will help you get stronger!

Every program you pick up and you try out, there should always be a why? Why are you doing this? What is the goal? When I started toying with the idea of this program I had been studying some theories from Juggernaut and their critiques of the Bulgarian system from Max's time he spent training with the Bulgarian coach and their team. I was also feeling very weak in my squat as I had been doing a ton of cardio and running. I wanted to get some strength back and I really just wanted to see what would happen if I worked up to a heavy squat everyday in a different format. Well, I got stronger! I was able to handle my 90% without a problem, but the big change was that I just felt overall stronger, not just in my squat but in my back and core and legs. No, my knees did not hurt, I kept the volume super low, I ate a ton of carbs, and I squatted!

The goal is to be able to come close to your max (about 90%), and for you to get use to pushing heavy weight often. The program starts with the first four weeks not wearing wraps or sleeves or a belt, this will promote strength of the joints and your core and back. We then finish up the program with two weeks wearing a belt and if you want sleeves or wraps you can wear them. After the first six weeks, the program spends two weeks as a "maintenance period" where you are only squatting three times a week with a little bit lower weight and a little bit higher volume, you can continue this maintenance period all the way through to your competition prep phase as this will allow you to put in more volume on your kettlebell days and allow you time for more cardio on the squat days. Check out the end of the book to see how I have continued this program for several months.

To start off we need your maxes on all your squats:

Back Squat   _____

Front Squat   _____

Overhead Squat   _____

Box Squat   _____

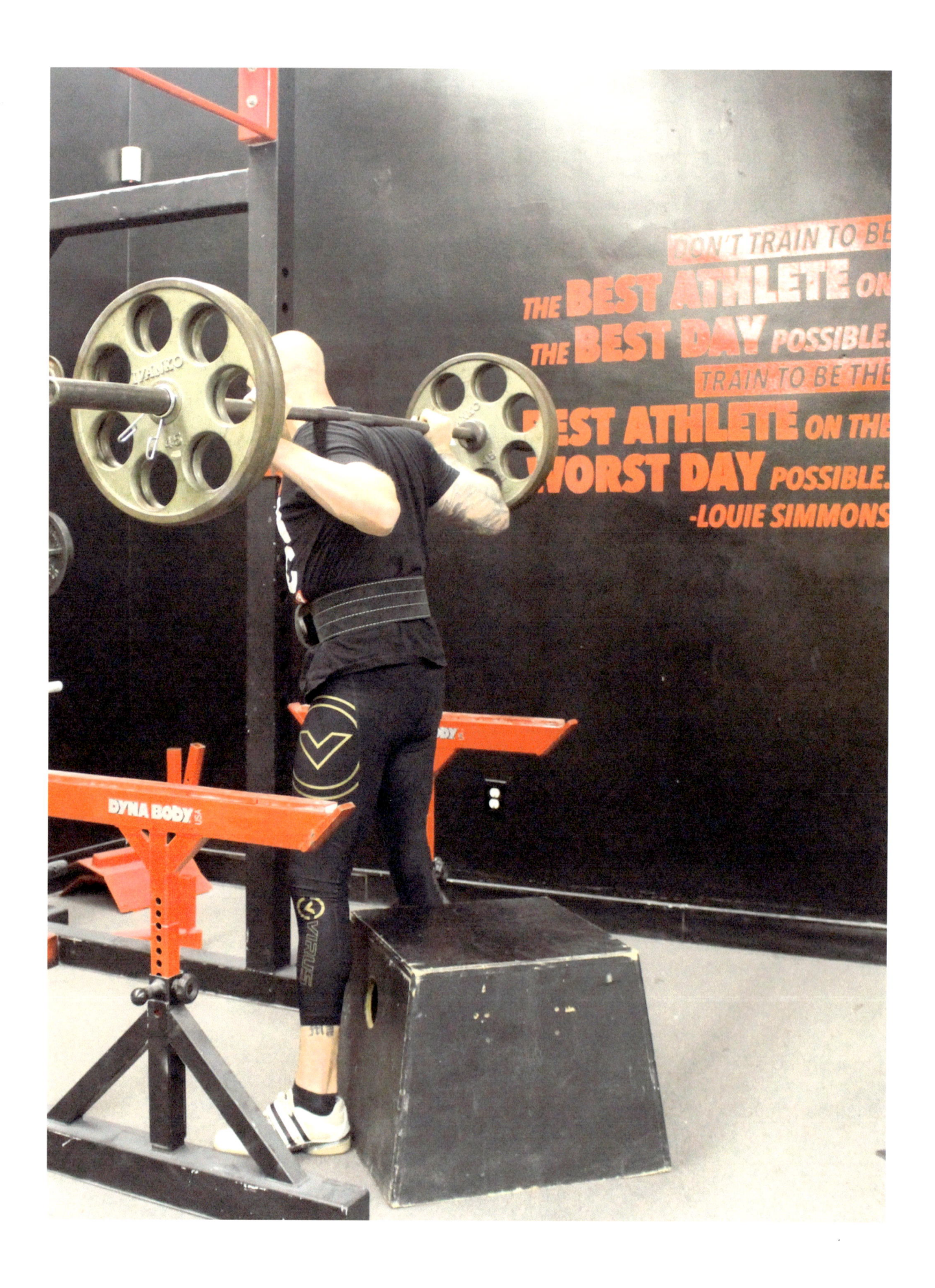

> DON'T TRAIN TO BE
> the BEST ATHLETE ON
> the BEST DAY POSSIBLE.
> TRAIN TO BE THE
> BEST ATHLETE ON THE
> WORST DAY POSSIBLE.
> —LOUIE SIMMONS

If your maxes are old, meaning you did them two years ago, don't use them, your maxes need to be within the last six months. If you have not hit a max on any of the lifts within the last six months, you will need to redo them, or I suggest taking 10% off your old maxes and use that number. As with most of this program, I like the 5-3-1 method, and you will see that format used in this program as well as using a similar format of 5-3-1-1 (not a Wendler 5-3-1 method as in first week is all 5 reps and second week is all 3 reps and third week is all 1 rep, no, I mean your rep schemes each day will be 5-3-1-1). Later in the maintenance phase you will be using a 5x1 format.

This program is not designed to get you a new one rep max! If you want to find a new one rep max after the first six weeks you can but I don't recommend it if you are prepping for a competition. This program is just designed to get your strength up before you start getting into more volume on kettlebell sport or powerlifting or any other strength sport you are involved in.

Each week the goal is to increase that heavy single by 5 to 10 pounds or by 2% to 2.25%. I recommend rounding down if you get a strange number on the percentage, we don't want any misses or failures! On the box squat we use slightly lower percentages because we are doing doubles and we want to promote more speed in the lift. Also on the overhead squat we use slightly lower numbers just for safety to prevent injury in this difficult and complex lift. On the cleans we use a lower percentage as we are doing several singles and we want to promote speed and explosiveness in this complex movement.

So if you are ready to get stronger, eat some oatmeal and some PB&J sandwiches and get ready to squat your ass off!!!

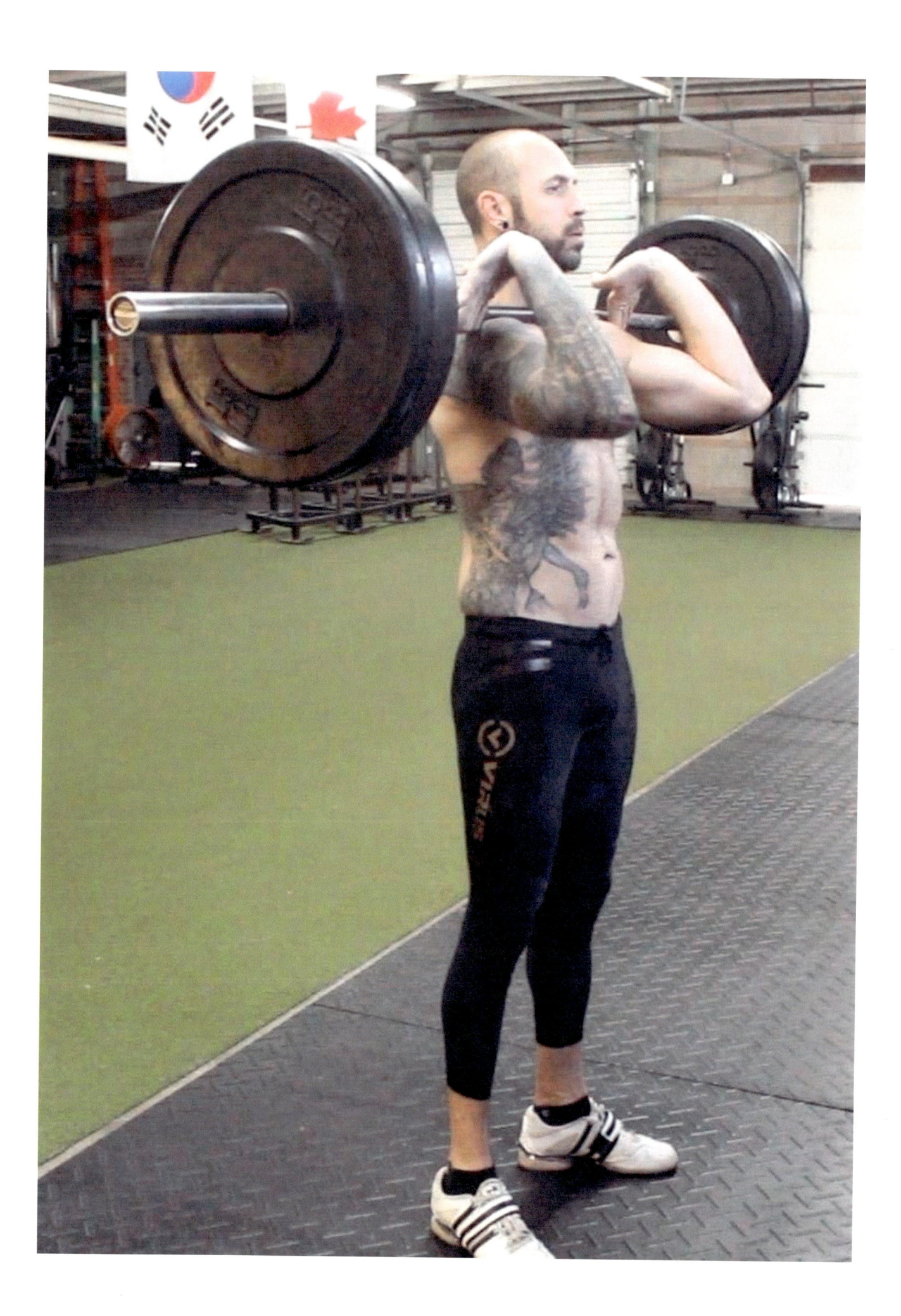

Monday – Front Squat

Base Max _____

Week 1

5 @ 55%_____ 3 @ 75%_____ 1 @ 80%_____

Week 2

5 @ 55%_____ 3 @ 75%_____ 1 @ 82%_____

Week 3

5 @ 60%_____ 3 @ 75%_____ 1 @ 84%_____

Week 4

5 @ 60%_____ 3 @ 75%_____ 1 @ 86%_____

Week 5

5 @ 65%_____ 3 @ 75%_____ 1 @ 88%_____

Week 6

5 @ 65%_____ 3 @ 75%_____ 1 @ 90%_____

*Front squats will continue in weeks 7 and 8 in the "Maintenance" section.

Tuesday – Squat Cleans

Base Max _____

Week 1

5 @ 50%_____   3 @ 55%_____   10x1 EMOM @ 60%_____

Week 2

5 @ 50%_____   3 @ 60%_____   10x1 EMOM @ 70%_____

Week 3

5 @ 60%_____   3 @ 70%_____   10x1 EMOM @ 75%_____

Week 4

5 @ 60%_____   3 @ 75%_____   10x1 EMOM @ 80%_____

Week 5

5 @ 60%_____   3 @ 75%_____   10x1 EMOM @ 82.5%_____

Week 6

5 @ 60%_____   3 @ 75%_____   10x1 EMOM @ 85%_____

*Cleans will not continue in weeks 7 and 8.

Wednesday – Back Squat

Base Max _____

Week 1

5 @ 55%_____   3 @ 75%_____   1 @ 80%_____

Week 2

5 @ 55%_____   3 @ 75%_____   1 @ 85%_____

Week 3

5 @ 55%_____   3 @ 80%_____   1 @ 87.5%_____

Week 4

5 @ 60%_____   3 @ 80%_____   1 @ 90%_____

Week 5

5 @ 65%_____   3 @ 85%_____   1 @ 92.5%_____

Week 6

5 @ 70%_____   3 @ 85%_____   1 @ 95%_____

*Back squats will continue in weeks 7 and 8 in the "Maintenance" section.

Thursday – Overhead Squat

Base Max _____

Week 1

5 @ 50%_____   3 @ 60%_____   1 @ 75%_____

Week 2

5 @ 50%_____   3 @ 60%_____   1 @ 80%_____

Week 3

5 @ 50%_____   3 @ 65%_____   1 @ 82%_____

Week 4

5 @ 55%_____   3 @ 65%_____   1 @ 85%_____

Week 5

5 @ 60%_____   3 @ 70%_____   1 @ 87.5%_____

Week 6

5 @ 60%_____   3 @ 70%_____   1 @ 90%_____

*Overhead squats will continue in weeks 7 and 8 in the "Maintenance" section.

Friday – Paused Back Squat

Base Max _____ (use your regular back squat max)

Week 1

5 @ 50%_____   3 @ 60%_____   1 @ 65%_____

Week 2

5 @ 50%_____   3 @ 60%_____   1 @ 70%_____

Week 3

5 @ 50%_____   3 @ 60%_____   1 @ 72.5%_____

Week 4

5 @ 55%_____   3 @ 65%_____   1 @ 75%_____

Week 5

5 @ 55%_____   3 @ 65%_____   1 @ 77.5%_____

Week 6

5 @ 60%_____   3 @ 70%_____   1 @ 80%_____

*Paused back squats will not continue in weeks 7 and 8.

Saturday – Box Squat with Chains
Chain weight – each side of the bar = 30 pounds guys / 15 pounds ladies

Base Max _____ (use your regular back squat max)

Week 1

5 @ 45%_____   3 @ 50%_____   5x2 @ 55%_____

Week 2

5 @ 50%_____   3 @ 55%_____   5x2 @ 60%_____

Week 3

5 @ 50%_____   3 @ 60%_____   5x2 @ 65%_____

Week 4

5 @ 50%_____   3 @ 60%_____   5x2 @ 67.5%_____

Week 5

5 @ 60%_____   3 @ 65%_____   5x2 @ 70%_____

Week 6

5 @ 60%_____   3 @ 70%_____   5x2 @ 75%_____

*Box squats will not continue in weeks 7 and 8.

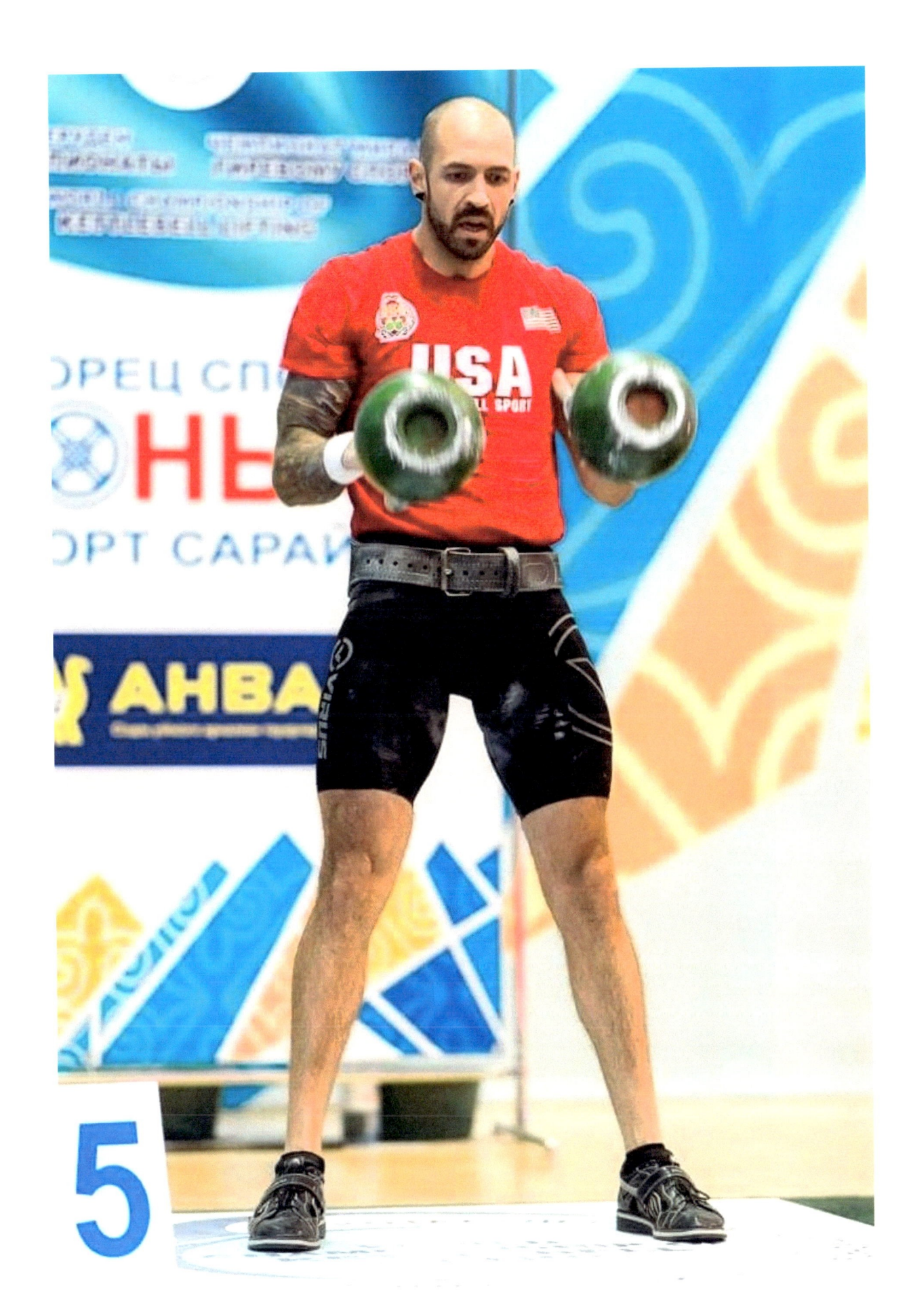

Maintenance

During maintenance weeks you will switch from squatting everyday to just three days a week, and you will squat on your off days from kettlebell training.

Tuesday – Front Squat – Base Max _____

Week 7

5 @ 55%_____   3 @ 87.5%_____   5x1 @ 90%_____

Week 8

5 @ 55%_____   3 @ 87.5%_____   5x1 @ 90%_____

Thursday – Overhead Squat – Base Max _____

Week 7

5 @ 55%_____   3 @ 87.5%_____   5x1 @ 80%_____

Week 8

5 @ 55%_____   3 @ 87.5%_____   5x1 @ 80%_____

Saturday – Back Squat – Base Max _____

Week 7

5 @ 55%_____   3 @ 87.5%_____   5x1 @ 90%_____

Week 8

5 @ 55%_____   3 @ 87.5%_____   5x1 @ 90%_____

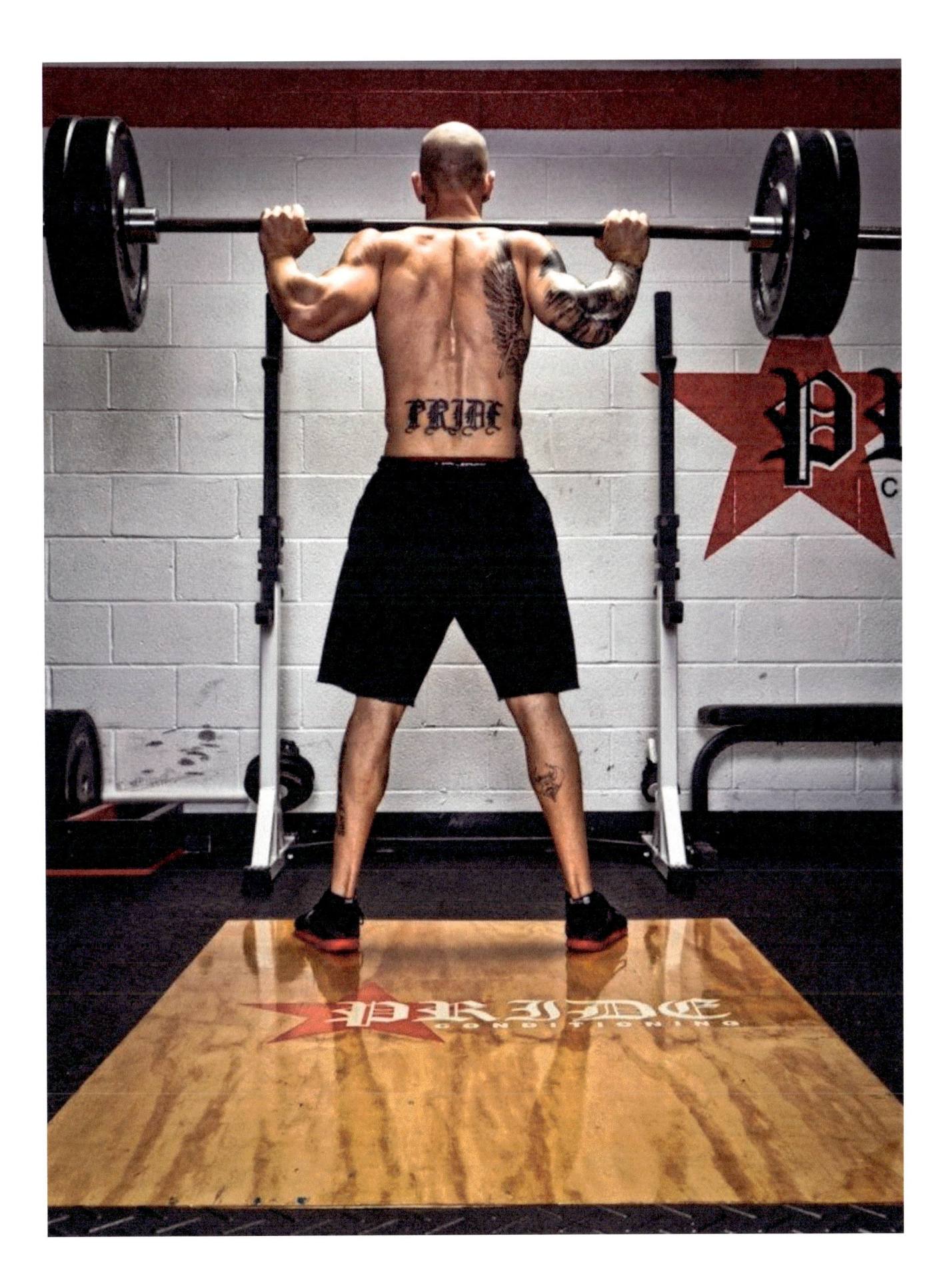

Conclusion

That is it! You are done! I hope you feel stronger and your lifts were all good!

If you are prepping for a competition it is probably time to start ramping up the volume in your training program and increasing your cardio work. I started this program right after I got back from nationals in August and I finished this program two months out from worlds in November. I continued the maintenance phase all the way through until three weeks out from leaving for South Korea. So I was on the maintenance phase for about six weeks and my body got very accustomed to hitting some squats and then going for a 3-4 mile run.

As always, if you have any questions please feel free to message me on facebook or instagram, or send me an email to info@prideconditioning.com. And if you need coaching or programming please email, I am always open to accepting new remote students into my program, just email me for pricing details. Thanks and good luck to you! PEACE!

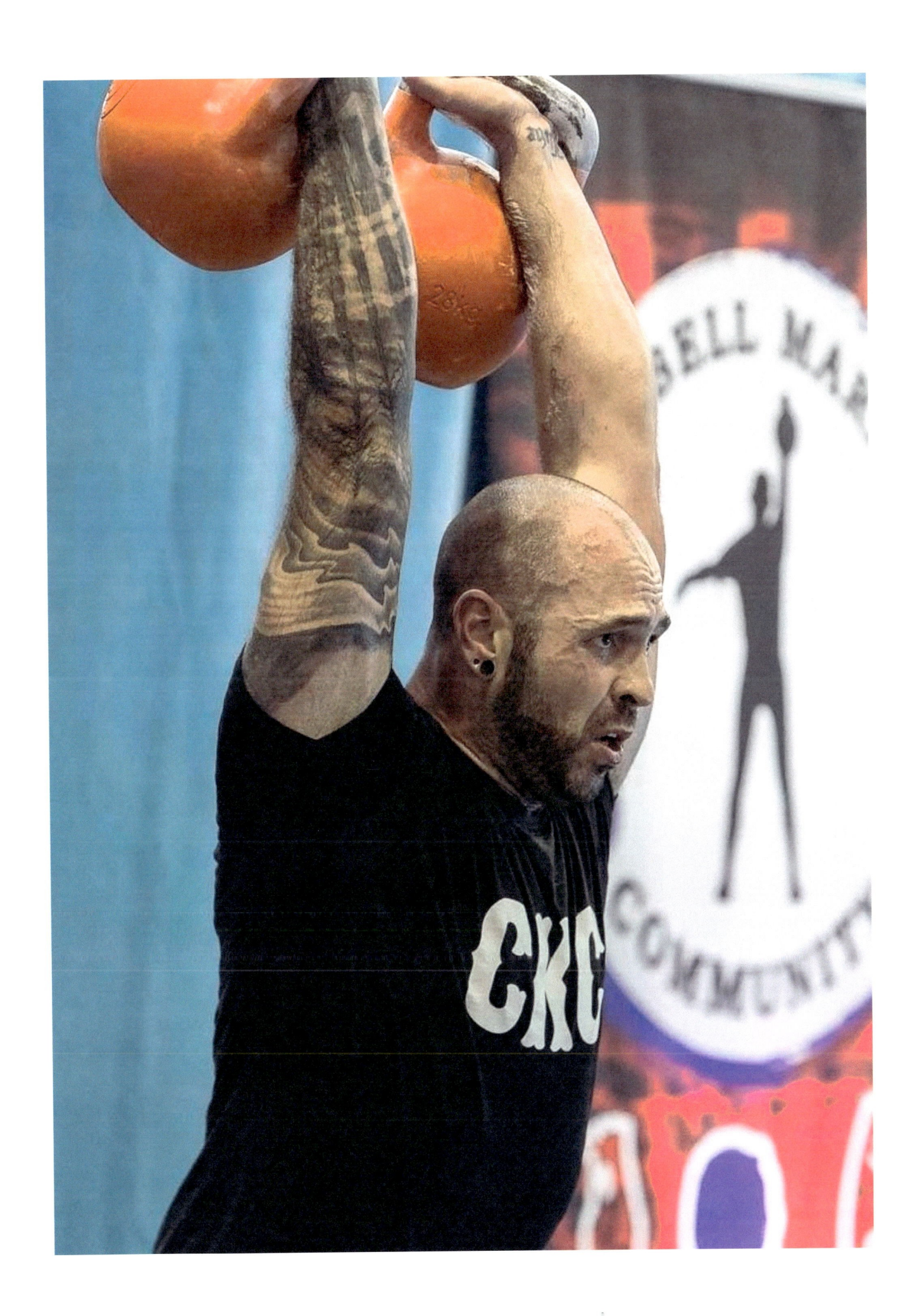

Bonus 6 Week Olympic Lifting Program

This book has actually been finished for many months, but I keep coming back to it thinking that there is something I am forgetting to tell you about, some information that I should be sharing with you, and finally six months later I realized what that is! I have been continuing to squat three days a week for almost a year after I first wrote and tested this program, and I am continually asked on social media and at competitions how I work powerlifting and Olympic lifting into my kettlebell schedule. I realized that this is the information I have been waiting to put into this book!

I am going to give you a six week Olympic lifting program you can follow after you finish the squat everyday program! You can actually repeat this six weeks over again two or three times as I have. After I finished the squat everyday program, I took some time off and then came back and got into some more Olympic lifting, then I went into competition training and then took some time off after that competition, and then I went into a 9 week box squat program (which I will be releasing for FREE through our website!!!). Once I was done with that box squat program I went into where I am now and that is a dedicated Olympic lifting plan with a very long term goal to get my clean and jerk to 225 and snatch to bodyweight.

This extra six week long Olympic lifting program is my extra gift to you! I was not planning to put it into this book but I feel it is good information for you to have, it is a small example of how I fit Olympic lifting in with Kettlebell, I will be releasing a much more in depth and detailed 12 week olifting and kettlebell program next year!

Six Week Basic Olympic Lifting and Kettlebell Program

Week 1

Monday
Front squat 5x5 @ 55%
Front squat drop set – drop by 10% and do 2 sets of 8 reps
Kettlebell - 2:00 doubles 4kg below comp weight
Kettlebell - 2:00/2:00 single arm at comp weight
Kettlebell - 2:00 doubles 2kg below comp weight

Tuesday
Oly - Snatch – Heavy singles from blocks
10x1 - 65%, 65%, 65%, 70%, 70%, 70%, 75%, 75%, 80%, 85%
Sled push – 10 x 50 feet @ 50% of back squat max

Wednesday
Kettlebell – Jerk – 20 rounds – 0:30 work – 1:30 rest – 8kg below comp weight
10 rounds – 3-6 Dips and 3-6 Pull ups and 10 back raises

Thursday
Oly - Clean and Jerk – Heavy singles from blocks
10x1 - 65%, 65%, 65%, 70%, 70%, 70%, 75%, 75%, 80%, 85%
Oly - Jerks (barbell) – from the rack or blocks – 6x – 2 push press + 1 Jerk @ 55%
Sled pull – 5:00 as many trips as possible at medium effort pace @ 50% of back squat

Friday
Back Squat – 5x5 @ 75% - set 5 drop by 15% and do 10 reps
Kettlebell - 5:00 – swing + long cycle – 4kg below comp weight

Saturday
Oly – max effort complex – 1 full clean, 1 hang clean, 1 front squat, 2 jerks
Oly – max effort complex – 2 hang squat snatch, 1 overhead squat
Kettlebell – Swing Snatch – 3:00/3:00 – 4kg below comp weight
Farmer carry – 5x1:00 – comp weight – rest as needed

Six Week Basic Olympic Lifting and Kettlebell Program

Week 2

Monday
Front squat 5x3 @ 60%
Front squat drop set – drop by 10% and do 2 sets of 7 reps
Kettlebell - 2:00 doubles 4kg below comp weight
Kettlebell - 2:00/2:00 single arm at comp weight
Kettlebell - 3:00 doubles 2kg below comp weight

Tuesday
Oly – Snatch – 8x – 1 snatch from floor + 1 snatch balance @ 70%
Sled push – 5x 1:00 work 2:00 rest

Wednesday
Kettlebell – Jerk ladder – doubles – 10 reps – start at 8kg under comp weight – 5 rounds up to comp weight – do the comp weight round twice – and then back down the ladder – rest until heart rate drops below 59%
10 rounds – 3-6 Dips and 3-6 Pull ups and 10 back raises * try to get one more rep than last week

Thursday
Oly - Clean – 6x2 @ 70% with 2 count pause on first dip
Oly - Jerk (barbell) – 6x2 @ 70% with 2 count pause on first dip
Sled pull – 6x 50 feet – load 75% of back squat max and take 10% off each trip

Friday
Back Squat – 5x3 @ 65%
Deadlift – 5x3 @ 65%
Kettlebell - 6:00 – 0:30 cleans – 0:30 jerks – 4kg below comp weight

Saturday
Oly – max effort complex – 1 full clean, 1 hang clean, 1 front squat, 1 jerk
Oly – max effort complex – 1 full snatch, 1 hang squat snatch, 1 overhead squat
Kettlebell – Snatch *This is one set no rest just switch hands* - comp weight
- Swing swing snatch 15/15
- Swing snatch 20/20
- Snatch 25/25

Single arm KB farmer carry, comp weight +2kg, 10x 0:30 each arm

Six Week Basic Olympic Lifting and Kettlebell Program

Week 3

Monday
Front squat 5x2 @ 70%
Front squat drop set – drop by 10% and do 2 sets of 6 reps
Kettlebell - 2:00 doubles 4kg below comp weight
Kettlebell - 1:00/1:00 single arm 2kg above comp weight
Kettlebell - 4:00 doubles 2kg below comp weight

Tuesday
Oly - Snatch – 6x1 from the floor @ 75%
Oly – Snatch - 5x2 power snatch from floor @ 50%-60%
Sled push

Wednesday
Kettlebell - Jerk ladder – doubles – 12 reps – start at 8kg under comp weight – 5 rounds up to comp weight – do the comp weight round twice – and then back down the ladder – rest until heart rate drops below 59%
10 rounds – 3-6 Dips and 3-6 Pull ups and 10 back raises * try to get one more rep than last week

Thursday
Oly - Clean – 6x1 from the floor @ 75% - 5x2 power clean from floor @ 50%-60%
Oly - Jerk (barbell) – 5x3 @ 75%
Sled pull

Friday
Back Squat – 5x3 @ 70%
Deadlift – 5x2 @ 70%
Kettlebell - 7:00 – 3 swings + 3 cleans + 3 jerks + 3 long cycle – 4kg below comp weight

Saturday
Oly – max effort complex – snatch pull to full snatch
Oly – max effort complex   1 full clean, 1 front squat, 1 jerk
Kettlebell – Snatch – 1:30/1:30 – 3 sets – comp weight, 2kg down, 4kg down

Six Week Basic Olympic Lifting and Kettlebell Program

Week 4

Monday
Front squat – 5x1 @ 75%
Front squat drop set – drop weight by 10% and do 2 sets of 5 reps
Kettlebell - Single arm – 5:00 – switch hands every 0:30 4kg above comp weight
Kettlebell - Doubles – 2:00 – comp weight
Kettlebell - Doubles – 1:00 – comp weight

Tuesday
Oly – Snatch – 5x - 1 hang power snatch + 1 full snatch from floor @ 75%-80%
Sled push – 6x 100 feet @ 50% of back squat max

Wednesday
Kettlebell - Jerk ladder – doubles – 15 reps – start at 8kg under comp weight – 5 rounds up to comp weight – do the top weight round twice – and then back down the ladder – rest until heart rate drops below 59%
10 rounds – 3-6 Dips and 3-6 Pull ups and 10 back raises * try to get one more rep than last week

Thursday
Oly – Clean – 5x - 1 hang power Clean + 1 full clean from floor @ 75%-80%
Oly – Jerk (barbell) – 3x1 @ 70%, 80%, 90% - 3x2 @ 70%
Sled pull – 3x - 2:00 work – 1:00 rest

Friday
Back Squat – 5x3 @ 75%
Deadlift – 5x1 @ 75%
Kettlebell - 8:00 – 1 swing + 2 cleans + 3 jerks – 4kg below comp weight

Saturday
Oly – max effort complex – 1 full snatch, 2 overhead squat
Oly – max effort complex – 2 full clean, 2 jerks
Kettlebell – Snatch *This is one set no rest just switch hands* - comp weight
- Swing swing snatch 20/20
- Swing snatch 25/25
- Snatch 30/30

Six Week Basic Olympic Lifting and Kettlebell Program

Week 5

Monday
Front squat – 3x1 @ 80%
Front squat drop set – drop weight by 10% and do 2 sets of 3 reps
Kettlebell - Single arm – 10:00 – switch hands every 1:00 4kg above comp weight

Tuesday
Oly - Power Snatch – 10x1 @ 65%
Sled push – 10 x 50 feet @ 50% of back squat max

Wednesday
Kettlebell – Jerk ladder – doubles - 10 reps – start at 8kg under comp weight – 6 rounds up to 2kg above comp weight – do the top weight round twice – and then back down the ladder – rest until heart rate drops below 59%
10 rounds – 3-6 Dips and 3-6 Pull ups and 10 back raises

Thursday
Oly - Clean – Heavy singles from blocks – 10x1 @ 75%-80%
Oly - Jerk (barbell) – from the rack or blocks – 6x – 2 push press + 1 Jerk @ 65%
Sled pull – 5:00 as many trips as possible at medium effort pace @ 50% of back squat

Friday
Back squat with pause – 5x2 @ 80%
Snatch grip deadlift – 5x3 @ 60% of max snatch
Kettlebell - 10:00 – slow long cycle (3 swings, 1 clean, 4 count hold in 4 positions) – 4kg below comp weight

Saturday
Oly – max effort complex – 2 full snatches
Oly – max effort complex – 2 full cleans, 1 jerk
Kettlebell – Snatches – 2:00/2:00 – 3 rounds – comp weight, 2kg down, 4kg down

Six Week Basic Olympic Lifting and Kettlebell Program

Week 6 – Deload & Maxout

Monday
Front squat – 2x1 @ 90%
Kettlebell LC – 20 rounds – 0:30 work – 1:00 rest – 6kg below comp weight – easy pace

Tuesday
Oly - Snatch – work up to your planned "opener" (around 90%)
Oly - Clean & Jerk – work up to your planned "opener" (around 90%)

Wednesday
Back Squat – 3x1 @ 80%
Kettlebell - Jerk – 10 rounds – 10 reps – 2kg below comp weight - rest until heart rate drops to to 59%

Thursday
Oly - Snatch – work up to your planned last warmup before opener (around 80%-85%)
Oly - Clean & Jerk – work up to your planned last warmup before opener (around 80%-85%)

Friday
"Rest" - go through snatch and clean & jerk movements with the bar and then do 3x2 on each movement with 40% of max

Saturday
Snatch to one rep max
3 @ 40%
2 @ 50%
2 @ 60%
1 @ 70%
1 @ 80%
1 @ 90%
1 @ 100%
1 @ 105%
…
Clean and Jerk to one rep max
2 @ 50%
2 @ 60%
1 @ 70%
1 @ 80%
1 @ 90%
1 @ 100%
1 @ 105%
…
Kettlebell – Swing Snatch – 4:00/4:00 – 4kg below comp weight

Made in the USA
Columbia, SC
23 October 2024